Name_____

Age_____

Start Weight_____

Goal Weight_____

Steps Per Day Goal_____

Calorie Goal Per Day_____

In This Food Logging Diary

1 Glass of Water = 250ml

1 of your 5 a Day = 80g of Fruit or Vegetables

Always Check The Labels, As some products will not count because of how they have been prepared.

30g of Dried Fruit

150ml Fruit Juice (only 1 counts)

Date___/___/___ Day of the Week M T W T F S S

Glasses of Water 1 2 3 4 5 6 7 8 + 1 of Your 5 a Day 1 2 3 4 5 +

Time	Meal Type	What Did You Have	Amount	Calories

 Weight   Total Steps   Total Calories

Date____/____/____ Day of the Week M T W T F S S

Glasses of Water 1 2 3 4 5 6 7 8 + 1 of Your 5 a Day 1 2 3 4 5 +

Time	Meal Type	What Did You Have	Amount	Calories

Weight   Total Steps   Total Calories

Date___/___/___ **Day of the Week** M T W T F S S

Glasses of Water 1 2 3 4 5 6 7 8 + 1 of Your 5 a Day 1 2 3 4 5 +

Time	Meal Type	What Did You Have	Amount	Calories

 Weight   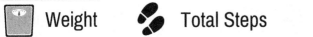 Total Steps   Total Calories

Date___/___/___ <u>Day of the Week</u> M T W T F S S

<u>Glasses of Water</u> 1 2 3 4 5 6 7 8 + <u>1 of Your 5 a Day</u> 1 2 3 4 5 +

Time	Meal Type	What Did You Have	Amount	Calories

Weight   Total Steps   Total Calories

Date___/___/___ Day of the Week M T W T F S S

Glasses of Water 1 2 3 4 5 6 7 8 + 1 of Your 5 a Day 1 2 3 4 5 +

Time	Meal Type	What Did You Have	Amount	Calories

 Weight 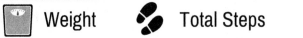 Total Steps 🔥 Total Calories

Date___/___/___ Day of the Week M T W T F S S

Glasses of Water 1 2 3 4 5 6 7 8 + 1 of Your 5 a Day 1 2 3 4 5 +

Time	Meal Type	What Did You Have	Amount	Calories

 Weight   Total Steps   Total Calories

Date___/___/___ Day of the Week M T W T F S S

Glasses of Water 1 2 3 4 5 6 7 8 + 1 of Your 5 a Day 1 2 3 4 5 +

Time	Meal Type	What Did You Have	Amount	Calories

 Weight   Total Steps   Total Calories

Date___/___/___ <u>Day of the Week</u> M T W T F S S

<u>Glasses of Water</u> 1 2 3 4 5 6 7 8 + <u>1 of Your 5 a Day</u> 1 2 3 4 5 +

Time	Meal Type	What Did You Have	Amount	Calories

Weight   Total Steps   Total Calories

Date___/___/___ Day of the Week M T W T F S S

Glasses of Water 1 2 3 4 5 6 7 8 + 1 of Your 5 a Day 1 2 3 4 5 +

Time	Meal Type	What Did You Have	Amount	Calories

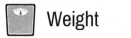 Weight Total Steps Total Calories

Date____/____/____ Day of the Week M T W T F S S

Glasses of Water 1 2 3 4 5 6 7 8 + 1 of Your 5 a Day 1 2 3 4 5 +

Time	Meal Type	What Did You Have	Amount	Calories

Weight   Total Steps   Total Calories

Date___/___/___ Day of the Week M T W T F S S

Glasses of Water 1 2 3 4 5 6 7 8 + 1 of Your 5 a Day 1 2 3 4 5 +

Time	Meal Type	What Did You Have	Amount	Calories

 Weight   Total Steps   Total Calories

Date___/___/___ Day of the Week M T W T F S S

Glasses of Water 1 2 3 4 5 6 7 8 + 1 of Your 5 a Day 1 2 3 4 5 +

Time	Meal Type	What Did You Have	Amount	Calories

 Weight 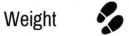 Total Steps Total Calories

Date___/___/___ Day of the Week M T W T F S S

Glasses of Water 1 2 3 4 5 6 7 8 + 1 of Your 5 a Day 1 2 3 4 5 +

Time	Meal Type	What Did You Have	Amount	Calories

 Weight   Total Steps   Total Calories

Date___/___/___ Day of the Week M T W T F S S

Glasses of Water 1 2 3 4 5 6 7 8 + 1 of Your 5 a Day 1 2 3 4 5 +

Time	Meal Type	What Did You Have	Amount	Calories

Weight   Total Steps   Total Calories

Date___/___/___ Day of the Week M T W T F S S

Glasses of Water 1 2 3 4 5 6 7 8 + 1 of Your 5 a Day 1 2 3 4 5 +

Time	Meal Type	What Did You Have	Amount	Calories

Weight   Total Steps   Total Calories

Date___/___/___ Day of the Week M T W T F S S

Glasses of Water 1 2 3 4 5 6 7 8 + 1 of Your 5 a Day 1 2 3 4 5 +

Time	Meal Type	What Did You Have	Amount	Calories

Weight   Total Steps   Total Calories

Date____/____/____ Day of the Week M T W T F S S

Glasses of Water 1 2 3 4 5 6 7 8 + 1 of Your 5 a Day 1 2 3 4 5 +

Time	Meal Type	What Did You Have	Amount	Calories

 Weight   Total Steps   Total Calories

Date___/___/___ <u>Day of the Week</u> M T W T F S S

<u>Glasses of Water</u> 1 2 3 4 5 6 7 8 + <u>1 of Your 5 a Day</u> 1 2 3 4 5 +

Time	Meal Type	What Did You Have	Amount	Calories

 Weight   Total Steps   Total Calories

Date___/___/___ Day of the Week M T W T F S S

Glasses of Water 1 2 3 4 5 6 7 8 + 1 of Your 5 a Day 1 2 3 4 5 +

Time	Meal Type	What Did You Have	Amount	Calories

Weight   Total Steps   Total Calories

Date___/___/___ <u>Day of the Week</u> M T W T F S S

<u>Glasses of Water</u> 1 2 3 4 5 6 7 8 + <u>1 of Your 5 a Day</u> 1 2 3 4 5 +

Time	Meal Type	What Did You Have	Amount	Calories

 Weight    Total Steps   Total Calories

Date___/___/___ <u>Day of the Week</u> M T W T F S S

<u>Glasses of Water</u> 1 2 3 4 5 6 7 8 + <u>1 of Your 5 a Day</u> 1 2 3 4 5 +

Time	Meal Type	What Did You Have	Amount	Calories

Weight   Total Steps   Total Calories

Date___/___/___ Day of the Week M T W T F S S

Glasses of Water 1 2 3 4 5 6 7 8 + 1 of Your 5 a Day 1 2 3 4 5 +

Time	Meal Type	What Did You Have	Amount	Calories

Weight   Total Steps   Total Calories

Date___/___/___ Day of the Week M T W T F S S

Glasses of Water 1 2 3 4 5 6 7 8 + 1 of Your 5 a Day 1 2 3 4 5 +

Time	Meal Type	What Did You Have	Amount	Calories

 Weight Total Steps Total Calories

Date___/___/___ Day of the Week M T W T F S S

Glasses of Water 1 2 3 4 5 6 7 8 + 1 of Your 5 a Day 1 2 3 4 5 +

Time	Meal Type	What Did You Have	Amount	Calories

 Weight   Total Steps   Total Calories

Date___/___/___ Day of the Week M T W T F S S

Glasses of Water 1 2 3 4 5 6 7 8 + 1 of Your 5 a Day 1 2 3 4 5 +

Time	Meal Type	What Did You Have	Amount	Calories

 Weight   Total Steps   Total Calories

Date____/____/____ Day of the Week M T W T F S S

Glasses of Water 1 2 3 4 5 6 7 8 + 1 of Your 5 a Day 1 2 3 4 5 +

Time	Meal Type	What Did You Have	Amount	Calories

Weight   Total Steps   Total Calories

Date___/___/___ Day of the Week M T W T F S S

Glasses of Water 1 2 3 4 5 6 7 8 + 1 of Your 5 a Day 1 2 3 4 5 +

Time	Meal Type	What Did You Have	Amount	Calories

Weight   Total Steps   Total Calories

Date___/___/___ <u>Day of the Week</u> M T W T F S S

<u>Glasses of Water</u> 1 2 3 4 5 6 7 8 + <u>1 of Your 5 a Day</u> 1 2 3 4 5 +

Time	Meal Type	What Did You Have	Amount	Calories

Weight   Total Steps   Total Calories

Date___/___/___ Day of the Week M T W T F S S

Glasses of Water 1 2 3 4 5 6 7 8 + 1 of Your 5 a Day 1 2 3 4 5 +

Time	Meal Type	What Did You Have	Amount	Calories

 Weight   Total Steps   Total Calories

Date___/___/___ <u>Day of the Week</u> M T W T F S S

<u>Glasses of Water</u> 1 2 3 4 5 6 7 8 + <u>1 of Your 5 a Day</u> 1 2 3 4 5 +

<u>Time</u>	<u>Meal Type</u>	<u>What Did You Have</u>	<u>Amount</u>	<u>Calories</u>

 Weight   Total Steps   Total Calories

Date___/___/___ Day of the Week M T W T F S S

Glasses of Water 1 2 3 4 5 6 7 8 + 1 of Your 5 a Day 1 2 3 4 5 +

Time	Meal Type	What Did You Have	Amount	Calories

 Weight   Total Steps   Total Calories

Date___/___/___ Day of the Week M T W T F S S

Glasses of Water 1 2 3 4 5 6 7 8 + 1 of Your 5 a Day 1 2 3 4 5 +

Time	Meal Type	What Did You Have	Amount	Calories

Weight   Total Steps   Total Calories

Date___/___/___ Day of the Week M T W T F S S

Glasses of Water 1 2 3 4 5 6 7 8 + 1 of Your 5 a Day 1 2 3 4 5 +

Time	Meal Type	What Did You Have	Amount	Calories

🔲 Weight   Total Steps   🔥 Total Calories

Date___/___/___ <u>Day of the Week</u> M T W T F S S

<u>Glasses of Water</u> 1 2 3 4 5 6 7 8 + <u>1 of Your 5 a Day</u> 1 2 3 4 5 +

<u>Time</u>	<u>Meal Type</u>	<u>What Did You Have</u>	<u>Amount</u>	<u>Calories</u>

Weight   Total Steps   Total Calories

Date___/___/___ Day of the Week M T W T F S S

Glasses of Water 1 2 3 4 5 6 7 8 + 1 of Your 5 a Day 1 2 3 4 5 +

Time	Meal Type	What Did You Have	Amount	Calories

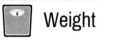 Weight   Total Steps   🔥 Total Calories

Date___/___/___ Day of the Week M T W T F S S

Glasses of Water 1 2 3 4 5 6 7 8 + 1 of Your 5 a Day 1 2 3 4 5 +

Time	Meal Type	What Did You Have	Amount	Calories

 Weight   Total Steps   Total Calories

Date____/____/____ __Day of the Week__ M T W T F S S

__Glasses of Water__ 1 2 3 4 5 6 7 8 + __1 of Your 5 a Day__ 1 2 3 4 5 +

Time	Meal Type	What Did You Have	Amount	Calories

 Weight   Total Steps   Total Calories

Date___/___/___ <u>Day of the Week</u> M T W T F S S

<u>Glasses of Water</u> 1 2 3 4 5 6 7 8 + <u>1 of Your 5 a Day</u> 1 2 3 4 5 +

Time	Meal Type	What Did You Have	Amount	Calories

 Weight Total Steps 🔥 Total Calories

Date___/___/___ Day of the Week M T W T F S S

Glasses of Water 1 2 3 4 5 6 7 8 + 1 of Your 5 a Day 1 2 3 4 5 +

Time	Meal Type	What Did You Have	Amount	Calories

Weight   Total Steps   Total Calories

Date___/___/___ Day of the Week M T W T F S S

Glasses of Water 1 2 3 4 5 6 7 8 + 1 of Your 5 a Day 1 2 3 4 5 +

Time	Meal Type	What Did You Have	Amount	Calories

Weight   Total Steps   Total Calories

Date___/___/___ Day of the Week M T W T F S S

Glasses of Water 1 2 3 4 5 6 7 8 + 1 of Your 5 a Day 1 2 3 4 5 +

Time	Meal Type	What Did You Have	Amount	Calories

 Weight   Total Steps   Total Calories

Date____/____/____ **Day of the Week** M T W T F S S

Glasses of Water 1 2 3 4 5 6 7 8 + 1 of Your 5 a Day 1 2 3 4 5 +

Time	Meal Type	What Did You Have	Amount	Calories

 Weight   Total Steps   Total Calories

Date___/___/___ Day of the Week M T W T F S S

Glasses of Water 1 2 3 4 5 6 7 8 + 1 of Your 5 a Day 1 2 3 4 5 +

Time	Meal Type	What Did You Have	Amount	Calories

 Weight   Total Steps   Total Calories

Date___/___/___ Day of the Week M T W T F S S

Glasses of Water 1 2 3 4 5 6 7 8 + 1 of Your 5 a Day 1 2 3 4 5 +

Time	Meal Type	What Did You Have	Amount	Calories

Weight   Total Steps   Total Calories

Date___/___/___ Day of the Week M T W T F S S

Glasses of Water 1 2 3 4 5 6 7 8 + 1 of Your 5 a Day 1 2 3 4 5 +

Time	Meal Type	What Did You Have	Amount	Calories

Weight   Total Steps   Total Calories

Date___/___/___ Day of the Week M T W T F S S

Glasses of Water 1 2 3 4 5 6 7 8 + 1 of Your 5 a Day 1 2 3 4 5 +

Time	Meal Type	What Did You Have	Amount	Calories

Weight   Total Steps   Total Calories

Date___/___/___ Day of the Week M T W T F S S

Glasses of Water 1 2 3 4 5 6 7 8 + 1 of Your 5 a Day 1 2 3 4 5 +

Time	Meal Type	What Did You Have	Amount	Calories

Weight   Total Steps   Total Calories

Date___/___/___ Day of the Week M T W T F S S

Glasses of Water 1 2 3 4 5 6 7 8 + 1 of Your 5 a Day 1 2 3 4 5 +

Time	Meal Type	What Did You Have	Amount	Calories

 Weight   Total Steps   Total Calories

Date___/___/___   Day of the Week M T W T F S S

Glasses of Water 1 2 3 4 5 6 7 8 +   1 of Your 5 a Day 1 2 3 4 5 +

Time	Meal Type	What Did You Have	Amount	Calories

 Weight   Total Steps   Total Calories

Date____/____/____ Day of the Week M T W T F S S

Glasses of Water 1 2 3 4 5 6 7 8 + 1 of Your 5 a Day 1 2 3 4 5 +

Time	Meal Type	What Did You Have	Amount	Calories

Weight   Total Steps   Total Calories

Date___/___/___ Day of the Week M T W T F S S

Glasses of Water 1 2 3 4 5 6 7 8 + 1 of Your 5 a Day 1 2 3 4 5 +

Time	Meal Type	What Did You Have	Amount	Calories

Weight   Total Steps   Total Calories

Date___/___/___ Day of the Week M T W T F S S

Glasses of Water 1 2 3 4 5 6 7 8 + 1 of Your 5 a Day 1 2 3 4 5 +

Time	Meal Type	What Did You Have	Amount	Calories

Weight   Total Steps   Total Calories

Date___/___/___ <u>Day of the Week</u> M T W T F S S

<u>Glasses of Water</u> 1 2 3 4 5 6 7 8 + <u>1 of Your 5 a Day</u> 1 2 3 4 5 +

Time	Meal Type	What Did You Have	Amount	Calories

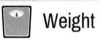 Weight   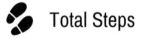 Total Steps   Total Calories

Date___/___/___ <u>Day of the Week</u> M T W T F S S

<u>Glasses of Water</u> 1 2 3 4 5 6 7 8 + <u>1 of Your 5 a Day</u> 1 2 3 4 5 +

Time	Meal Type	What Did You Have	Amount	Calories

 Weight   Total Steps   Total Calories

Date ___/___/___ Day of the Week M T W T F S S

Glasses of Water 1 2 3 4 5 6 7 8 + 1 of Your 5 a Day 1 2 3 4 5 +

Time	Meal Type	What Did You Have	Amount	Calories

 Weight   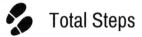 Total Steps   Total Calories

Date___/___/___ Day of the Week M T W T F S S

Glasses of Water 1 2 3 4 5 6 7 8 + 1 of Your 5 a Day 1 2 3 4 5 +

Time	Meal Type	What Did You Have	Amount	Calories

Weight　　　Total Steps　　　Total Calories

Date ___/___/___ Day of the Week M T W T F S S

Glasses of Water 1 2 3 4 5 6 7 8 + 1 of Your 5 a Day 1 2 3 4 5 +

Time	Meal Type	What Did You Have	Amount	Calories

Weight   Total Steps   Total Calories

Date___/___/___ Day of the Week M T W T F S S

Glasses of Water 1 2 3 4 5 6 7 8 + 1 of Your 5 a Day 1 2 3 4 5 +

Time	Meal Type	What Did You Have	Amount	Calories

Weight   Total Steps   Total Calories

Date ___ / ___ / ___ Day of the Week M T W T F S S

Glasses of Water 1 2 3 4 5 6 7 8 + 1 of Your 5 a Day 1 2 3 4 5 +

Time	Meal Type	What Did You Have	Amount	Calories

 Weight   Total Steps   Total Calories

Date ___/___/___ Day of the Week M T W T F S S

Glasses of Water 1 2 3 4 5 6 7 8 + 1 of Your 5 a Day 1 2 3 4 5 +

Time	Meal Type	What Did You Have	Amount	Calories

 Weight　　　 Total Steps　　　 Total Calories

Date___/___/___ <u>Day of the Week</u> M T W T F S S

<u>Glasses of Water</u> 1 2 3 4 5 6 7 8 + <u>1 of Your 5 a Day</u> 1 2 3 4 5 +

Time	Meal Type	What Did You Have	Amount	Calories

 Weight   Total Steps   Total Calories

Date___/___/___ Day of the Week M T W T F S S

Glasses of Water 1 2 3 4 5 6 7 8 + 1 of Your 5 a Day 1 2 3 4 5 +

Time	Meal Type	What Did You Have	Amount	Calories

Weight   Total Steps   Total Calories

Date___/___/___ <u>Day of the Week</u> M T W T F S S

<u>Glasses of Water</u> 1 2 3 4 5 6 7 8 + <u>1 of Your 5 a Day</u> 1 2 3 4 5 +

Time	Meal Type	What Did You Have	Amount	Calories

 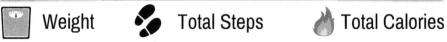

Weight   Total Steps   Total Calories

Date___/___/___ <u>Day of the Week</u> M T W T F S S

<u>Glasses of Water</u> 1 2 3 4 5 6 7 8 + <u>1 of Your 5 a Day</u> 1 2 3 4 5 +

Time	Meal Type	What Did You Have	Amount	Calories

Weight   Total Steps   Total Calories

Date___/___/___ Day of the Week M T W T F S S

Glasses of Water 1 2 3 4 5 6 7 8 + 1 of Your 5 a Day 1 2 3 4 5 +

Time	Meal Type	What Did You Have	Amount	Calories

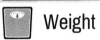 Weight   Total Steps   Total Calories

Date___/___/___ **Day of the Week** M T W T F S S

Glasses of Water 1 2 3 4 5 6 7 8 + **1 of Your 5 a Day** 1 2 3 4 5 +

Time	Meal Type	What Did You Have	Amount	Calories

 Weight   Total Steps   Total Calories

Date___/___/___ Day of the Week M T W T F S S

Glasses of Water 1 2 3 4 5 6 7 8 + 1 of Your 5 a Day 1 2 3 4 5 +

Time	Meal Type	What Did You Have	Amount	Calories

 Weight   Total Steps   Total Calories

Date___/___/___ <u>Day of the Week</u> M T W T F S S

<u>Glasses of Water</u> 1 2 3 4 5 6 7 8 + <u>1 of Your 5 a Day</u> 1 2 3 4 5 +

Time	Meal Type	What Did You Have	Amount	Calories

 Weight Total Steps 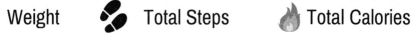 Total Calories

Date ___ / ___ / ___ Day of the Week M T W T F S S

Glasses of Water 1 2 3 4 5 6 7 8 + 1 of Your 5 a Day 1 2 3 4 5 +

Time	Meal Type	What Did You Have	Amount	Calories

 Weight   Total Steps   Total Calories

Date___/___/___ Day of the Week M T W T F S S

Glasses of Water 1 2 3 4 5 6 7 8 + 1 of Your 5 a Day 1 2 3 4 5 +

Time	Meal Type	What Did You Have	Amount	Calories

 Weight   Total Steps   Total Calories

Date___/___/___ <u>Day of the Week</u> M T W T F S S

<u>Glasses of Water</u> 1 2 3 4 5 6 7 8 + <u>1 of Your 5 a Day</u> 1 2 3 4 5 +

Time	Meal Type	What Did You Have	Amount	Calories

 Weight   Total Steps Total Calories

Date ___ / ___ / ___ Day of the Week M T W T F S S

Glasses of Water 1 2 3 4 5 6 7 8 + 1 of Your 5 a Day 1 2 3 4 5 +

Time	Meal Type	What Did You Have	Amount	Calories

 Weight   Total Steps   Total Calories

Date___/___/___ Day of the Week M T W T F S S

Glasses of Water 1 2 3 4 5 6 7 8 + 1 of Your 5 a Day 1 2 3 4 5 +

Time	Meal Type	What Did You Have	Amount	Calories

 Weight   Total Steps   Total Calories

Date____/____/____ <u>Day of the Week</u> M T W T F S S

<u>Glasses of Water</u> 1 2 3 4 5 6 7 8 + <u>1 of Your 5 a Day</u> 1 2 3 4 5 +

Time	Meal Type	What Did You Have	Amount	Calories

Weight   Total Steps   Total Calories

Date___/___/___ Day of the Week M T W T F S S

Glasses of Water 1 2 3 4 5 6 7 8 + 1 of Your 5 a Day 1 2 3 4 5 +

Time	Meal Type	What Did You Have	Amount	Calories

Weight   Total Steps   Total Calories

Date___/___/___ <u>Day of the Week</u> M T W T F S S

<u>Glasses of Water</u> 1 2 3 4 5 6 7 8 + <u>1 of Your 5 a Day</u> 1 2 3 4 5 +

<u>Time</u>	<u>Meal Type</u>	<u>What Did You Have</u>	<u>Amount</u>	<u>Calories</u>

Weight   Total Steps   Total Calories

Date___/___/___ <u>Day of the Week</u> M T W T F S S

<u>Glasses of Water</u> 1 2 3 4 5 6 7 8 + <u>1 of Your 5 a Day</u> 1 2 3 4 5 +

Time	Meal Type	What Did You Have	Amount	Calories

 Weight   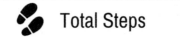 Total Steps   Total Calories

Date___/___/___ <u>Day of the Week</u> M T W T F S S

<u>Glasses of Water</u> 1 2 3 4 5 6 7 8 + <u>1 of Your 5 a Day</u> 1 2 3 4 5 +

Time	Meal Type	What Did You Have	Amount	Calories

 Weight   Total Steps   Total Calories

Date___/___/___ **Day of the Week** M T W T F S S

Glasses of Water 1 2 3 4 5 6 7 8 + 1 of Your 5 a Day 1 2 3 4 5 +

Time	Meal Type	What Did You Have	Amount	Calories

 Weight   Total Steps   Total Calories

Date____/____/____ **Day of the Week** M T W T F S S

Glasses of Water 1 2 3 4 5 6 7 8 + **1 of Your 5 a Day** 1 2 3 4 5 +

Time	Meal Type	What Did You Have	Amount	Calories

Weight   Total Steps   Total Calories

Date___/___/___ <u>Day of the Week</u> M T W T F S S

<u>Glasses of Water</u> 1 2 3 4 5 6 7 8 + <u>1 of Your 5 a Day</u> 1 2 3 4 5 +

Time	Meal Type	What Did You Have	Amount	Calories

 Weight   Total Steps   Total Calories

Date___/___/___ Day of the Week M T W T F S S

Glasses of Water 1 2 3 4 5 6 7 8 + 1 of Your 5 a Day 1 2 3 4 5 +

Time	Meal Type	What Did You Have	Amount	Calories

 Weight   Total Steps   Total Calories

Date___/___/___ <u>Day of the Week</u> M T W T F S S

<u>Glasses of Water</u> 1 2 3 4 5 6 7 8 + <u>1 of Your 5 a Day</u> 1 2 3 4 5 +

<u>Time</u>	<u>Meal Type</u>	What Did You Have	<u>Amount</u>	<u>Calories</u>

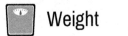 Weight   Total Steps   Total Calories

Date___/___/___ Day of the Week M T W T F S S

Glasses of Water 1 2 3 4 5 6 7 8 + 1 of Your 5 a Day 1 2 3 4 5 +

Time	Meal Type	What Did You Have	Amount	Calories

 Weight   Total Steps   Total Calories

Date___/___/___ Day of the Week M T W T F S S

Glasses of Water 1 2 3 4 5 6 7 8 + 1 of Your 5 a Day 1 2 3 4 5 +

Time	Meal Type	What Did You Have	Amount	Calories

Weight   Total Steps   Total Calories

Date_____/_____/_____   Day of the Week M T W T F S S

Glasses of Water 1 2 3 4 5 6 7 8 +   1 of Your 5 a Day 1 2 3 4 5 +

Time	Meal Type	What Did You Have	Amount	Calories

 Weight   Total Steps   Total Calories

Date____/____/____ Day of the Week M T W T F S S

Glasses of Water 1 2 3 4 5 6 7 8 + 1 of Your 5 a Day 1 2 3 4 5 +

Time	Meal Type	What Did You Have	Amount	Calories

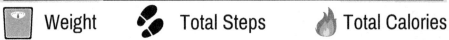 Weight   Total Steps   Total Calories

Date___/___/___ Day of the Week M T W T F S S

Glasses of Water 1 2 3 4 5 6 7 8 + 1 of Your 5 a Day 1 2 3 4 5 +

Time	Meal Type	What Did You Have	Amount	Calories

 Weight   Total Steps   🔥 Total Calories

Date___/___/___ <u>Day of the Week</u> M T W T F S S

<u>Glasses of Water</u> 1 2 3 4 5 6 7 8 + <u>1 of Your 5 a Day</u> 1 2 3 4 5 +

<u>Time</u>	<u>Meal Type</u>	<u>What Did You Have</u>	<u>Amount</u>	<u>Calories</u>

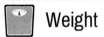 Weight Total Steps Total Calories

Date___/___/___ <u>Day of the Week</u> M T W T F S S

<u>Glasses of Water</u> 1 2 3 4 5 6 7 8 + <u>1 of Your 5 a Day</u> 1 2 3 4 5 +

Time	Meal Type	What Did You Have	Amount	Calories

 Weight 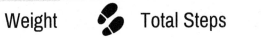 Total Steps Total Calories

Date___/___/___ <u>Day of the Week</u> M T W T F S S

<u>Glasses of Water</u> 1 2 3 4 5 6 7 8 + <u>1 of Your 5 a Day</u> 1 2 3 4 5 +

Time	Meal Type	What Did You Have	Amount	Calories

 Weight   Total Steps   Total Calories

Date___/___/___   <u>Day of the Week</u> M T W T F S S

<u>Glasses of Water</u> 1 2 3 4 5 6 7 8 + <u>1 of Your 5 a Day</u> 1 2 3 4 5 +

Time	Meal Type	What Did You Have	Amount	Calories

Weight   Total Steps   Total Calories

Date___/___/___ Day of the Week M T W T F S S

Glasses of Water 1 2 3 4 5 6 7 8 + 1 of Your 5 a Day 1 2 3 4 5 +

Time	Meal Type	What Did You Have	Amount	Calories

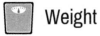 Weight   Total Steps   Total Calories

Date___/___/___ Day of the Week M T W T F S S

Glasses of Water 1 2 3 4 5 6 7 8 + 1 of Your 5 a Day 1 2 3 4 5 +

Time	Meal Type	What Did You Have	Amount	Calories

Weight   Total Steps   Total Calories

Date___/___/___ Day of the Week M T W T F S S

Glasses of Water 1 2 3 4 5 6 7 8 + 1 of Your 5 a Day 1 2 3 4 5 +

Time	Meal Type	What Did You Have	Amount	Calories

Weight   Total Steps   Total Calories

Date____/____/____ <u>Day of the Week</u> M T W T F S S

<u>Glasses of Water</u> 1 2 3 4 5 6 7 8 + <u>1 of Your 5 a Day</u> 1 2 3 4 5 +

Time	Meal Type	What Did You Have	Amount	Calories

 Weight   Total Steps   Total Calories

Date___/___/___ Day of the Week M T W T F S S

Glasses of Water 1 2 3 4 5 6 7 8 + 1 of Your 5 a Day 1 2 3 4 5 +

Time	Meal Type	What Did You Have	Amount	Calories

 Weight   Total Steps   Total Calories

Date_____/_____/_____ Day of the Week M T W T F S S

Glasses of Water 1 2 3 4 5 6 7 8 + 1 of Your 5 a Day 1 2 3 4 5 +

Time	Meal Type	What Did You Have	Amount	Calories

 Weight Total Steps Total Calories

Date___/___/___ Day of the Week M T W T F S S

Glasses of Water 1 2 3 4 5 6 7 8 + 1 of Your 5 a Day 1 2 3 4 5 +

Time	Meal Type	What Did You Have	Amount	Calories

Weight   Total Steps   Total Calories

Printed in Great Britain
by Amazon

39781002R00056